Paleo Diet for Triathletes

Delicious Paleo Diet Plan, Recipes and Cookbook Designed to Support the Specific Needs of Triathletes - from Sprint to Ironman and Beyond (Food for Fitness Series)

Lars Andersen

Published by Nordic Standard Publishing

Atlanta, Georgia USA

NORDICSTANDARD
PUBLISHING

ISBN 978-1-484145-22-7

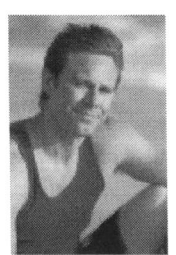

Lars Andersen (signature)

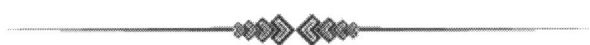

What Our Readers Are Saying

"Detailed and easy to follow. I would definitely recommend this book to fellow triathletes"

★★★★★ **Victor A. Saylor (Hallsville, OH)**

"Precisely the type of guide I'd been hunting (and gathering) for!"

★★★★☆ **Leila L. Hutchinson (San Diego, CA)**

"Really interesting adaption of the Paleo diet especially for endurance athletes"

★★★★☆ **Timothy V. Bruno (Palmyra, VA)**

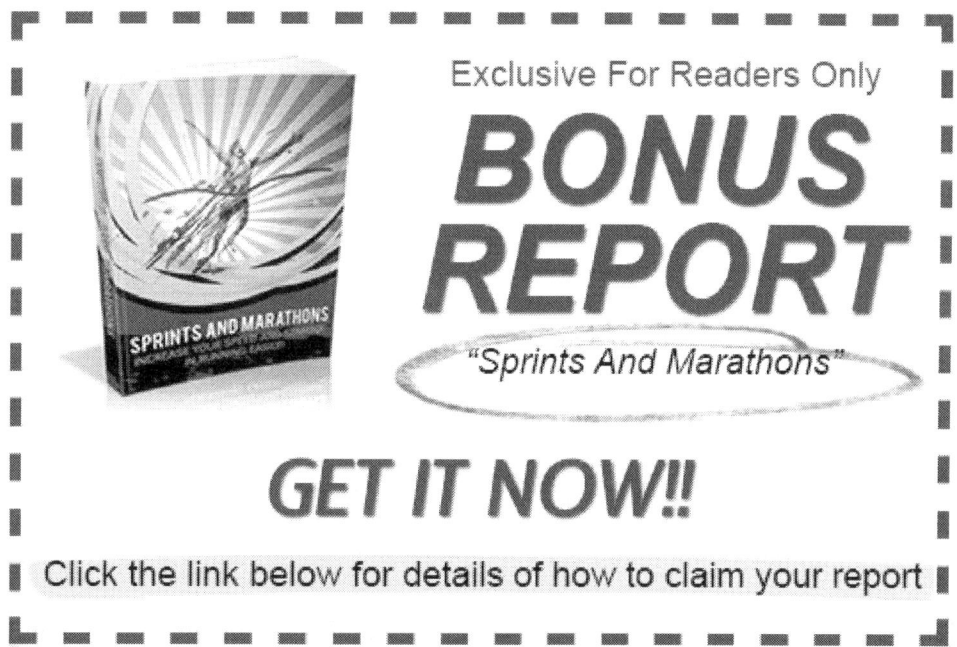

Exclusive Bonus Download: Sprints And Marathons

Sure-fire Ways To Master Your Running Efforts!

This Book Is One Of The Most Valuable Resources In The World When It Comes To Getting Serious Results In Your Life!

Running is the act by which animals, including human beings, move by the power of the feet. Speeds may vary and range from jogging to a sprint. A lot of individuals compete in track events that place participants in a contest to test speed in a sprint or endurance in a marathon. The running mechanics are the same, but additional factors are very different in a marathon versus a sprint.

Consider this...

Whether your goal is to determine a fresh personal record in your next 5k, win your age bracket at the following charity run or qualify for a state or national contest, you may learn to run faster.

Are you ready?

Introducing... Sprints And Marathons

This powerful tool will provide you with everything you need to know to be a success and achieve your goal.

Who Can Use This Book?

- Life Coaches
- Runners
- Personal Development Enthusiasts
- Self Improvement Bloggers
- Business owners
- Internet marketers
- Network marketers
- Web Publishers
- Writers and Content Creators
- And Many More!

Go to the end of this book for the download link for this Bonus!

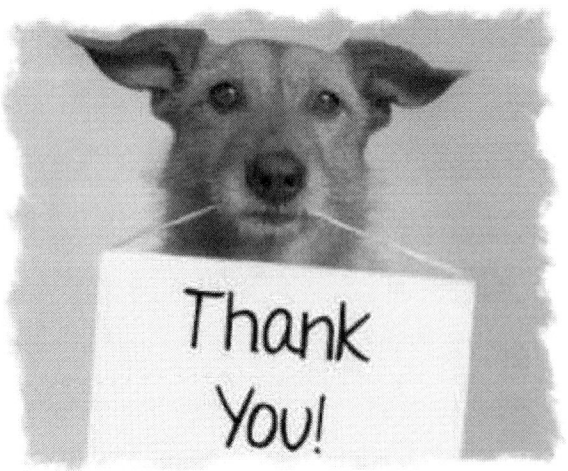

Thank you for downloading my book. Please REVIEW this book on Amazon. I need your feedback to make the next edition better. Thank you so much!

Books by Lars Andersen

The Smoothies for Runners Book

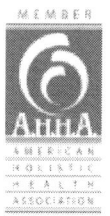

Table of Contents

Disclaimer

Paleo Diet for Triathletes

"Vegetarians are cool. All I eat are vegetarians – except for the occasional mountain lion steak" – Ted Nugent

The Paleo diet, also known as the caveman diet, is the common name given to the Paleolithic diet. In essence, it's based on the diet of our hunter-gatherer ancestors some 2.5 million years ago in the Paleolithic Era and revolves around eating foods which occur naturally and avoiding foods which would be unrecognizable to a Paleolithic caveman! A popular rule of thumb proposed by Paleo advocates is, "If it's in a box, you shouldn't be eating it."

The current US Department of Agriculture (USDA) healthy eating guidelines promote a balanced daily diet consisting of 60 percent carbohydrates, 30 percent fats, and 10 percent protein. Switching from USDA recommendations to a Paleo diet will generally lead to an increase in your overall protein and fat intake and a drop in your overall carbohydrate intake. At first glance, this appears to go against current sports nutritional advice which promotes carbohydrates as "the athlete's best friend" and the main source of fuel for sports activities. However, Paleo sources of fuel are *quality* sources, with healthful carbohydrates coming from fruits and vegetables; protein coming from lean meats with low levels of saturated fat and fish with high levels of omega-3 essential fatty acids; and fats coming from natural, unprocessed oils and "fatty" foodstuffs.

Cutting all "modern" foodstuffs from your diet, including all forms of grain as well as highly processed convenience foods, leaves a diet of all natural foodstuffs, for example:

- **Meat** – grass-fed rather than grain-fed animal sources.
- **Fowl** – chicken, turkey, duck, and game birds.
- **Fish** – wild fish rather than farmed fish as the latter can contain unhealthy levels of mercury and other toxins.
- **Eggs**
- **Vegetables** – excluding modern farmed varieties.
- **Oils** – any natural source such as olive oil, coconut oil, walnut oil, or avocado oil.
- **Fruits** – berries in particular and other fruits in moderation.
- **Nuts** – excluding peanuts.
- **Tubers** – sweet potatoes and yams in particular.

There is no *one* Paleo diet, and it's important to note that a Paleo-based diet is not necessarily a "low-carb diet" as such. Some hunter-gatherer populations would have survived and thrived on a low-carb diet; others would have lived equally well on a high-carb diet of fish, tubers, and coconut. An important element of all Paleo-based diets is that locally sourced organic produce should make up the bulk of your daily food intake whenever possible. However, this can prove expensive in some areas of today's world, so aiming to eat the best quality produce you can afford is an important step in terms of getting the most from a Paleo diet.

All You Can Eat!

The basic principle behind a Paleo diet is to eat only natural foodstuffs and to effectively eat all you want! There's no calorie counting or portion control required and in terms of eating a Paleo diet to fuel and maximize your swimming, cycling and running performance, it's all about tailoring your carbohydrate intake to match your activity levels. If you are in serious training for a long-distance competitive event, your need for "starchy" carbohydrate fuel may increase in comparison to fuelling your body for shorter distance or less competitive activities. The most common sources of starchy carbs for Paleo triathletes are sweet potato and potato, although rice and quinoa may be included on occasion when energy demands are high.

Paleo Fuel Sources

Paleo "purists" eat only foods which can be hunted, fished or gathered. Foods include meat, offal, seafood, eggs, insects, fruits, nuts, seeds, vegetables, mushrooms, herbs and spices. Excluded foods include grains, legumes – beans and peanuts – dairy products, refined sugar, salt and processed oils. However, other Paleo-based diets include "modern" foods which were not available to our cavemen ancestors but support the macronutrient composition of a Paleolithic diet none-the-less. These foods include milk and dairy products, rice, potatoes and some processed oils such as olive oil or canola oil.

Protein

Meat sources:

    Beef – with the exception of fiber, beef contains most of the nutrients your body needs:

- Calcium- essential for strong bones and teeth, and plays an important role in nerve transmission and muscle functions.
- Vitamin C – needed to make collagen, a protein essential for healthy gums, teeth, bones, cartilage and skin. Also aids the absorption of iron from plant food and is an important antioxidant. Antioxidants protect against free radicals, potentially harmful chemicals which are formed by your body as a by-product of its metabolic processes.
- Folate – needed for the formation of proteins in the body.
- Iron – an essential component of hemoglobin, the oxygen carrying pigment in red blood cells, and also important in energy metabolism.
- Iodine – vital for the production of thyroid hormones which govern the efficiency of converting food into energy.
- Manganese – a vital component of many enzymes involved in energy production.
- Zinc – vital for normal growth and development, and plays an important role in the functioning of the immune system.
- Selenium – an antioxidant which protects against free radical damage.
- Chromium – monitors blood sugar levels and stimulates glucose uptake in cells. Also helps to control fat and cholesterol levels in the blood.
- Fluoride – plays a role in protecting tooth enamel against the acids which may cause decay.
- Silicon – required for strong, flexible joints and connective tissues.

The vitamin and mineral content of beef depends on the soil grazed. Grass-fed beef provides far greater health benefits than grain-fed beef. Lean beef contains less than five percent fat, half of which is saturated fat.

Lamb – provides a rich source of protein, B vitamins, zinc and iron.

Pork – one of the leanest meat sources of protein; lower in fat than beef and lamb. A useful source of zinc and iron and an excellent source of B vitamins:

- B vitamins – play an important role in releasing energy from food.
- Vitamin B12 – essential for all growth and division of cells, and for red cell formation.

Offal – ox liver and calves' liver are rich sources of easily absorbed iron. Also:

- Vitamin A – needed for normal cell division and growth, and plays an important role in maintaining the mucous membranes of the respiratory, digestive and urinary tracts.
- Vitamin B12

Kidneys also provide a rich source of B12 and both liver and kidney are low in fat.

Game and Game Birds – provide excellent sources of protein, with a much lower fat content than domesticated animals such as chicken. This category includes sources such as venison, rabbit, wild boar and pheasant. They offer a rich source of B vitamins and iron, also:

- Potassium – essential for the transmission of all nerve impulses, and works in conjunction with sodium to maintain a healthy fluid and electrolyte balance within the cells. Electrolytes are charged particles that circulate in the blood, helping to regulate the body's fluid balance.
- Phosphorus – essential for the absorption of many nutrients, and plays a vital role in the release of energy in cells.

Wild game, when available, represents a chemical free source of protein compared to farmed game, but sources must always be sustainable.

Other animal sources:

Fish – all forms of fish provide excellent sources of protein, however, wild varieties offer healthier options than farmed versions. This also applies to **seafood**, with organic sources of crab, oysters, shrimp, scallops, lobster mussels and clams representing healthier choices.

- **Oysters** – excellent source of zinc and copper, needed for healthy bone and connective tissue growth. Copper also helps the body to absorb iron from food and is present in many enzymes which protect against free radical damage.
- **Mussels** – rich source of iron and iodine.
- **Scallops** – rich source of selenium.

- **Crab** – good source of potassium and zinc; also contains magnesium, which assists in nerve impulses and is important for muscle contraction.
- **Shrimps** – rich source of iodine; also useful source of selenium and calcium.
- **Clams** – excellent source of iron and useful source of zinc.

Eggs – omega-3 enriched eggs offer an excellent source of protein and healthy fat; a large egg contains around 6-8 grams of protein and 5-7 grams of fat, around 2 grams of which is saturated fat. However, it's recommended that no more than six eggs should be consumed per week due to the high cholesterol content. A rich source of:

- Vitamin B12
- Choline (in yolks) – aids the transport of cholesterol in the blood and plays an important role in fat metabolism.

Plant sources:

Hemp – provides a good source of protein, a healthy balance of omega-3 and omega-6 essential fatty acids, and contains many B vitamins, vitamin A, calcium and iron. Also:

- Vitamin D – needed to absorb calcium and phosphorus.
- Vitamin E – an important antioxidant.
- Sodium – essential for nerve and muscle function, and works in conjunction with potassium to regulate the body's fluid balance.
- And dietary fiber.

Green leafy vegetables – greens provide a good source of plant protein along with many other health benefits:

- **Beet greens** – the leafy tops of beets contain calcium, iron and beta-carotene, a powerful antioxidant. Research has also found that consuming beets on a regular basis can enhance an athlete's tolerance to high-intensity exercise.
- **Collard greens** – a good source of omega-3 essential fatty acids which have anti-inflammatory properties.
- **Lettuce** – a good source of vitamin C, beta-carotene, folate, calcium and iron.
- **Mustard greens** – an excellent source of antioxidant vitamins A, C, E, and vitamin K which plays an essential role in the formation of certain proteins. Also contains carotenes and flavonoids which are powerful antioxidants, and calcium, iron, magnesium, potassium, zinc, selenium and manganese.
- **Swiss chard** – a rich source of vitamin A, C and K, B vitamins, omega-3 fatty acids, and a number of antioxidants and flavonoids. Also contains copper, calcium, sodium, potassium, iron, manganese and phosphorus.
- **Turnip greens** – a rich source of beta-carotene, vitamin C, and a useful source of folate.
- **Spinach** – a rich source of carotenoids, including antioxidants beta-carotene and lutein. Also contains vitamin C and potassium.

Cruciferous vegetables

- **Cabbage** - rich source of vitamin C, vitamin K, and a good source of vitamin E, potassium and beta-carotene. Vitamin K is essential in the formation of many proteins - the body's building blocks - and vitamin E has an important role to play in preventing free radical damage.
- **Broccoli** - another rich source of vitamin C. Broccoli also contains beta-carotene, iron and potassium, and is high in bioflavonoids and other antioxidants. Iron is essential for the production of hemoglobin, the oxygen carrying pigment in red blood cells, and myoglobin, a similar pigment which stores oxygen in your muscles.
- **Kale** - a good source of iron, calcium, vitamin C and beta-carotene.
- **Cauliflower** – a rich source of vitamin C.
- **Rutabaga** – a good source of vitamin A and iron.
- **Kohlrabi** – a good source of vitamin C, calcium, phosphorus and iron.
- **Watercress** – rich source of vitamin C, beta-carotene and iron.

Fats

Not all fats are equal. Like carbohydrates, fats also provide energy. In fact, fats yield nine calories per gram compared to only four calories per gram for carbohydrates. However, fat is a much slower source of energy so when you are training hard, your body relies on your glycogen stores to fuel your performance by providing a faster release of energy. All carbohydrates are converted to glycogen and stored in your body. During longer duration, steadier-paced training sessions or events, your body aims to conserve as much of its glycogen reserves as possible by using some of its fat stores for energy instead.

Good quality fat sources in a Paleo-based diet are the saturated fats provided by grass-fed meat and the fat provided by organic eggs. The preferred cooking fats are tallow, lard, grass-fed butter, ghee, coconut oil, palm oil and occasionally olive oil, although processed oils should be avoided whenever possible and used for dressing foods rather than cooking foods. Some oils contain high levels of omega-6 fatty acids which can cause an inflammatory response in your body. For this reason, most nut and seed oils should be used sparingly. Macadamia nuts offer the lowest levels of omega-6 but alternatives include flax seed oil (linseed oil), walnut oil, canola and avocado oil. Avocados themselves are a rich source of healthy fat, with one fruit containing as many as 400 healthful calories.

Your body can make its own fat from excess carbohydrates and protein in your diet but it cannot manufacture certain essential unsaturated fats, meaning that the foods you eat are your body's only supply. The essential fatty acids are omega-3, found in green leafy vegetables and some vegetable oils, and omega-6, found in vegetable oils such as olive oil and sunflower oil. Creating a healthy omega-6 and omega-3 balance with a ratio of 2:1 or 1:1 brings optimum benefits in terms of overall health and wellbeing. Fats act as a carrier for fat-soluble vitamins, including vitamins A, D, K, and E, and they provide insulation and protection for your body.

Many nuts and seeds provide excellent sources of fat and also protein. Good Paleo choices include:

- **Flax seeds** - also known as linseeds, provide a good source of protein and are high in omega-3 essential fatty acids. They also contain B vitamins which are involved in the release of energy from food.

- **Pumpkin seeds** – a rich source of protein and fat along with numerous vitamins and minerals including B vitamins, vitamin E, copper, manganese, potassium, calcium, magnesium, iron, zinc and selenium. Copper is present in many enzymes which protect against free radicals and helps the body to absorb iron from food.
- **Sunflower seeds** – provide protein along with vitamin E, selenium, magnesium and copper.
- **Almonds** – provide protein along with calcium, magnesium, potassium, vitamin E and other antioxidants. They may also help to relieve leg cramps, including night cramps, a common complaint in endurance sports. Leg cramps are the result of fatigue and an electrolyte imbalance. Eating almonds or making an almond butter using organic, grass-fed butter is an effective way to restore and then maintain the balance when in hard training.
- **Cashews** – a good source of protein and rich in iron, phosphorus, selenium, zinc and magnesium.
- **Walnuts** – provide protein and also a rich source of omega-3 fatty acids.

Adding oils to raw foods or foods after cooking as a dressing is a practical way to boost your healthy fat intake. Popular choices include olive oil and coconut oil. The "healthy" saturated fat content of coconut oil provides energy-giving calories and many other health benefits including anti-inflammatory properties.

Carbohydrates

Paleo carbohydrate sources are mainly fruits and vegetables. Carbohydrates can be split into two main categories: simple carbohydrates or **sugars**, and complex carbohydrates or **starches**. Starches provide a much slower release of energy compared to sugars, making them the preferred source of fuel for multi-sport and long-distance activities. The natural sugar content of most fruits means they must be consumed in moderation to avoid sugar "spikes" and "crashes" whereas the majority of vegetables can be consumed on an "all you can eat" basis.

Good sources of Paleo carbohydrate include:

- **Cassava** – a good source of "starchy" carbohydrate. Also provides calcium, iron, manganese, phosphorus, potassium, B vitamins, vitamin C and dietary fiber. Cassava flour is gluten-free.
- **Taro root** – a starchy vegetable offering a rich source of potassium, and a useful source of calcium, vitamins C and E, B vitamins, manganese, magnesium and copper. Taro leaves are also relatively high in protein.
- **Plantains** – a good low sugar source of starchy carbohydrate, also an excellent source of potassium and dietary fiber, and a useful source of vitamins A and C.
- **Yam** – a good source of vitamin B6, vitamin C, potassium and manganese.
- **White potatoes** – a good source of starchy carbohydrate, protein and fiber. They also provide vitamin C and potassium.
- **Sweet potatoes** – a good source of vitamin B6, vitamin C, vitamin D, iron, magnesium, potassium and beta-carotene.
- **Squash** – a good source of vitamins C and A, and also a useful source of calcium and iron.

In moderation, the following fruits also provide a good source of carbohydrate:

- **Strawberries** - a rich source of vitamin C and also an aid to the absorption of iron from vegetables.

- **Pears** - a good source of vitamin C, potassium, pectin and bioflavonoids. Pectin provides fiber, and bioflavonoids are powerful antioxidants.
- **Mangoes** - a good source of vitamin C and beta-carotene.
- **Bananas** - a rich source of potassium.
- **Apple** – offers a small amount of vitamin C.
- **Peach** – a good source of vitamins A and C.
- **Blueberries** - often described as "the ultimate brain food," blueberries have an antioxidant content of around five times higher than other fruits and vegetables. Research has discovered that a daily serving of 100 grams can stimulate new brain cell growth and slow down the effects of mental ageing. Mental sharpness can provide a "winning edge" in competitive triathlon events.

Both fruits and vegetables provide a healthful source of carbohydrates for energy but the added fiber content of vegetables helps to slow the absorption of sugar and thereby a slower and steadier release of energy is provided. Dark green leafy vegetables are nutritionally dense, making them an ideal source of energy to fuel endurance sports such as triathlon.

Performance Fuel

All carbohydrates are converted into glucose and glycogen before they can be used to fuel everyday activities and exercise. While swimming, cycling and running, the working muscles are fuelled by glucose in the blood, and by glycogen from stores in the liver and in the muscles. Glucose and glycogen are inter-convertible. When the body has a sufficient supply of glucose, carbohydrates are converted to glycogen and stored, but if glucose is in short supply, glycogen is converted to glucose ready for use.

During endurance sports, the body conserves as much of its glycogen reserves as possible by using some of its fat stores for energy. However, compared to carbohydrate, fat is a very slow source of energy, meaning that as the intensity of the exercise increases, the body switches to using glycogen to provide a faster release of energy. Your body can only store a limited amount of glycogen, with the muscles able to store enough for up to around two hours of intense exercise. After exercising, your body's ability to store glycogen is elevated. This period of around 30 minutes is known as the "glycogen window" and consuming appropriate foods in this window helps replenish glycogen stores, promote muscle repair and restoration, and thereby aid recovery after a long or intense training session.

Carbohydrates are crucial to achieving a top endurance performance and replenishing glycogen stores after training is essential if energy levels are to be maintained. Eating a Paleo-based meal containing a mix of carbohydrates and protein is an ideal post-training source of energy-replenishing nutrients but it's not always possible to prepare or eat a full meal within the 30-minute glycogen window after a ride. A snack containing starchy carbohydrates such as potatoes or sweet potatoes prepared in advance can be a practical way to bridge the gap between finishing a ride and sitting down to eat a full meal. A green smoothie made with green, leafy vegetables and berries blended with water provides a convenient and nutritious alternative. If you choose to include some dairy products in your Paleo diet, adding milk or yogurt to a post-ride smoothie can boost the protein content. Milk contains whey protein which is fast-acting and helps to reduce the effects of muscle damage immediately after an intense ride, and casein protein which is slow-acting and helps to continue the repair process long after the ride.

The only way to improve your performance as a triathlete is to train your body appropriately. The foods you eat provide your body with fuel for training, they *do not* improve your swim, cycle or run times on their own! Quality is more important than quantity in triathlon training terms. Shorter and more intense sessions, including interval sessions in all three disciplines and hill work on foot and on your bike, are an important element of a performance training program, even for long-distance events. The quality foods you eat provide quality fuel for your body, allowing you to put in a quality effort in every training session. However, it's also crucial to remember the importance of rest and recovery. Active recovery sessions at less than 75 percent of your maximum heart rate pace not only allow your body to regenerate after intense training, they maximize your body's use of fat as its main source of energy.

Flavorsome Fuel

The list of non-Paleo foods to avoid often seems much longer than the list of foods which *can* be eaten when choosing to follow a Paleo-based diet. However, as just one example, a Paleo meal could be grass-fed lamb broiled with a hint of rosemary and served with chard sautéed in bacon ends. That's flavorsome fuel! If you need additional carbohydrates to fuel intensive training, adding potatoes smothered in grass-fed butter to your plate is a tasty way to meet those needs.

The use of fresh herbs and spices can add a flavorsome twist to your meals or to a green smoothie with the additional benefit of boosting the nutritional content. Popular choices include:

- **Parsley** - one cup of parsley contains 2 grams of protein. It is also rich in calcium and provides iron, copper, magnesium, potassium, zinc, phosphorus, beta-carotene and vitamin C.
- **Dill** – adds a sweet flavor to foods and contains calcium, iron, manganese, vitamin C, and beta-carotene.
- **Sorrel** - provides iron, magnesium and calcium.
- **Basil** - provides beta-carotene, iron, potassium, copper, manganese and magnesium
- **Coriander** - provides a mild, peppery flavor along with anti-inflammatory properties, vitamin C, iron and magnesium.
- **Ginger** - research has found that ginger can be helpful in reducing muscle aches after intense exercise.
- **Garlic** - contains antiviral and antibacterial properties.
- **Turmeric** - contains antibacterial, antibiotic and anti-inflammatory properties. It also adds a vibrant yellow color!
- **Nutmeg** - adds richness and warmth to vegetable dishes. Works particularly well with cauliflower.
- **Cayenne** - a rich source of vitamin A.
- **Black pepper** - contains iron, beta-carotene, vitamin C and bioflavonoids.

Other Paleo sources of nutrition and flavor include:

- **Bell peppers**
- **Eggplants**
- **Mushrooms**
- **Onions**
- **Radishes**
- **Tomatillos**
- **Cucumber**

- And if you have a sweet tooth, **raspberries** or **Brazil nuts** covered in **organic dark chocolate** make a delicious treat!

Many Paleo advocates believe that all caffeine sources, including chocolate, should be avoided but others include organic, high cocoa content varieties in moderation, along with coffee and tea when prepared without the addition of sugar.

5 Steps to Paleo Powered Performance

A Paleo-based diet is essentially a diet which revolves around consuming moderate amounts of meat, moderate amounts of fruit and unlimited amounts of vegetables.

Becoming a Paleo-fuelled triathlete can be summarized as follows:

- **Eat only real food** – buy locally grown, fresh, organic produce whenever possible.
- **Do not eat any processed or refined carbohydrates** – avoid sugar, flour, pasta, bread and candy. Eat fruits for sweet flavors or honey occasionally if your activity levels require an extra energy boost.
- **Eat plenty of high quality fat** – sources include meat, eggs, avocado and also dairy if you choose to include it. Avoid processed oils and industrial meats, and eat nuts in moderation to help keep a healthy omega-6:3 balance.
- **Eat only high quality meat** – buy grass-fed or wild sources whenever possible; organ meats provide cost-effective sources of quality protein.
- **Tailor your non-refined carbohydrate intake to match your activity levels** – eat as many vegetables as you like, potatoes and sweet potatoes in moderation, rice or quinoa only when energy demands are high, and avoid all grains containing gluten.

Paleo Recipes – Triathletes

Breakfast

Strawberry smoothie

Preparation time	5 minutes
Ready time	5 minutes
Serves	4
Serving quantity/unit	350 G / 12 ounces
Calories	268 Cal
Total Fat	14g
Cholesterol	0mg
Sodium	109mg
Total Carbohydrates	36g
Dietary fibers	6g
Sugars	27g
Protein	4g
Vitamin C	1.42
Vitamin A	0.08
Iron	0.07
Calcium	0.05

Ingredients

- 3 cup of organic almond milk
- 4 cup of strawberries
- 3 tbsps. of flax seed
- ½ cup of pecan nuts
- 3 tbsps. of raw honey

Method

- Combine all the ingredients in a food processor and pulse until smooth.

Bell pepper and mushroom casserole

Preparation time	15 minutes
Ready time	50 minutes
Serves	4
Serving quantity/unit	160 G / 5 ounces
Calories	116 Cal
Total Fat	6 g
Cholesterol	207 mg
Sodium	384 mg
Total Carbohydrates	7 g
Dietary fibers	1g
Sugars	4g
Protein	9g
Vitamin C	0.55
Vitamin A	0.17
Iron	0.07
Calcium	0.08

Ingredients

- 1 cup of mushrooms, chopped
- ½ cup of green bell pepper, chopped
- ½ cup of red bell pepper, chopped
- 1 onion, finely chopped
- 5 organic eggs, beaten
- ½ cup of grass fed milk (or almond milk)
- 1 tbsp. of parsley, finely chopped
- ½ tsp. of salt
- ½ tsp. of pepper

Method

- Preheat oven to 350°F.
- Cook the vegetables in a non-stick pan over medium heat for 4-5 minutes or until tender. Drain and pour into a baking dish.
- Stir eggs, milk, salt, pepper and parsley until blended.
- Pour over the vegetables in the baking dish and bake for 30-35 minutes or until a fork inserted in the center comes out clean.

Banana Pancake

Preparation time	15 minutes
Ready time	30 minutes
Serves	4
Serving quantity/unit	151 G / 5 ounces
Calories	336 Cal
Total Fat	24 g
Cholesterol	85mg
Sodium	44mg
Total Carbohydrates	23g
Dietary fibers	6g
Sugars	10 g
Protein	12g
Vitamin C	0.09
Vitamin A	0.04
Iron	0.11
Calcium	0.14

Ingredients

- 2 organic eggs
- 1 ½ cup of almond meal
- 2 medium bananas
- ½ cup of grass-fed milk or almond milk
- 1 tbsp. of coconut oil, melted

Method

- Pre-heat a non-stick pan.
- Mash the bananas and combine with the eggs, milk and almond flour in a large bowl mixing until the batter is smooth.
- Brush the pan with the coconut oil and pour in ¼ to 1/3 of batter, cook for 2 or 3minutes, until bubbles burst on the surface, turn and cook the other side for 1 minute or until golden.
- Serve immediately.

Pumpkin and apricot bread

Preparation time	20 minutes
Ready time	60 minutes
Serves	6
Serving quantity/unit	100 G / 4 ounces
Calories	328 Cal
Total Fat	23 g
Cholesterol	82 mg
Sodium	358 mg
Total Carbohydrates	27g
Dietary fibers	4g
Sugars	21g
Protein	8g
Vitamin C	0
Vitamin A	0.54
Iron	0.1
Calcium	0.08

Ingredients

- 1 ½ cup of almond meal
- 1 tsp. of baking soda
- 1 tsp. of pumpkin spice
- ½ cup of organic pumpkin puree
- 1/3 cup of raw honey
- ¼ cup of coconut oil, melted
- 3 organic eggs
- ¼ cup of dried apricots, finely sliced

Method

- Preheat oven to 350F.
- Combine the almond meal, baking soda and spices in a food processor, add the pumpkin puree, raw honey, oil and eggs to the flour mixture and pulse until the batter is homogenous.
- Add the apricots and scoop batter into a small, non-stick, loaf pan.
- Bake for 35-40 minutes or until a toothpick comes out clean.

Apricot, coconut and almond squares

Preparation time	15 minutes
Ready time	35 minutes
Serves	6
Serving quantity/unit	59 G / 2 ounces / 1 square
Calories	216 Cal
Total Fat	19 g
Cholesterol	0mg
Sodium	3mg
Total Carbohydrates	10g
Dietary fibers	3g
Sugars	4g
Protein	6g
Vitamin C	0.04
Vitamin A	0.1
Iron	0.07
Calcium	0.07

Ingredients

- 1 ¼ cup of almonds
- ½ cup of dried coconut chips
- 1 cup of dried apricots
- 1 tbsp. of coconut oil, melted
- 2 tbsp. of almond butter

Method

- Preheat oven to 350°F.
- Pulse almonds in a food processor until very finely chopped. Set aside.
- Combine dried apricots, coconut oil and almond butter in a food processor and pulse until a homogenous paste is formed.
- Combine the apricot paste with the almonds in a large bowl and add the coconut. Mix until well blended.
- Press the batter into a small square/rectangular baking pan previously lined with non-stick baking paper.
- Bake for 15-20 minutes. Let cool and cut into squares.

Crepes with fresh blackberry syrup

Preparation time	15 minutes
Ready time	45 minutes
Serves	4
Serving quantity/unit	210 G / 7 ounces / 2 crepes
Calories	370 Cal
Total Fat	30g
Cholesterol	205mg
Sodium	86mg
Total Carbohydrates	21g
Dietary fibers	6g
Sugars	15g
Protein	11g
Vitamin C	0.28
Vitamin A	0.08
Iron	0.15
Calcium	0.08

Ingredients

Crepes:

- 5 organic eggs
- ¾ cup of coconut milk
- 1/3 cup of almond meal
- 1/3 cup of coconut flakes
- 1+1 tbsps. of coconut oil, melted

- Blackberry syrup:
- 2 cup of blackberries
- 4 tbsps. of water
- 2 tbsps. of raw honey

Method

Crepes:

- Pre-heat a non-stick pan.
- Pulse the coconut flakes and the almond meal in a food processor until very fine flour is formed.
- Combine the eggs, milk, and one tablespoon of oil in a large bowl and mix until the batter is homogenous. Add the almond and coconut flour and whisk until the batter is smooth.
- Brush the pan with the remaining coconut oil and pour in ¼ of batter.
- Gently tilt the pan until the surface is evenly covered with batter and cook for 1 or 2 minutes, until golden.
- Turn and cook the other side.

Blackberry syrup:

- Combine the blackberries and water in a medium saucepan and bring to a simmer.
- Simmer 10-15 minutes or until the blackberries are soft and the syrup thickens, add the raw honey and remove from heat.
- Serve the crepes still warm with the blackberry syrup.

Baked apple

Preparation time	10 minutes
Ready time	1h10
Serves	4
Serving quantity/unit	240 G / 8 ounces / 2 apples
Calories	271 Cal
Total Fat	0g
Cholesterol	0 mg
Sodium	3 mg
Total Carbohydrates	75g
Dietary fibers	13g
Sugars	57g
Protein	1g
Vitamin C	0.69
Vitamin A	0
Iron	0.27
Calcium	0.06

Ingredients

- 8 apples, cored
- 8 tsps. of raw honey
- 2 tbsps. of water
- 8 tbsps. of raisins (unsweetened)
- 8 tsps. of cinnamon

Method

- Preheat oven to 350 °F (175°C).
- Place the apple in a baking dish and fill each core with one tablespoon of raisins and one teaspoon of cinnamon.
- Stir together the honey and water and pour the mixture over the apples.
- Bake for 1 hour basting every 15-20 minutes with the juices.

Snack

Blackberry and raisins squares

Preparation time	10 minutes
Ready time	30 minutes
Serves	8
Serving quantity/unit	60 G / 8 ounces
Calories	180 Cal
Total Fat	13g
Cholesterol	21 mg
Sodium	12mg
Total Carbohydrates	15 g
Dietary fibers	3g
Sugars	9 g
Protein	4g
Vitamin C	0.05
Vitamin A	0.01
Iron	0.07
Calcium	0.06

Ingredients

- ¾ cup of almonds
- ¾ cup of dried coconut chips
- 1 tbsp. of flax seed
- 3 tbsps. of water
- 2 tbsps. of raw honey
- 3 tbsp. of almond butter
- 1 tbsp. of grass-fed milk or almond milk

- 1 organic egg
- ¾ cup of blackberries
- ¼ cup of raisins (unsweetened)

Method

- Preheat oven to 350F.
- Pulse the flax seeds in a food processor until grind, transfer into a small bowl and add two tablespoons of water. Set aside.
- Pulse the almonds, and coconut chips in a food processor until very finely chopped.
- Combine the raw honey, almond butter, egg, flax seed mixture and milk in a large bowl and mix until well blended. Add the almond mixture and mix. Finally, fold in the blackberries and raisins.
- Press the batter into a small square/rectangular baking pan previously lined with non-stick baking paper.
- Bake for 15-20 minutes. Let cool and cut into squares.

Kale chips

Preparation time	5 minutes
Ready time	20 minutes
Serves	4
Serving quantity/unit	90 G / 3 ounces
Calories	160 Cal
Total Fat	15 g
Cholesterol	0 mg
Sodium	321 mg
Total Carbohydrates	8 g
Dietary fibers	1g
Sugars	0 g
Protein	3g
Vitamin C	1.36
Vitamin A	2.06
Iron	0.07
Calcium	0.1

Ingredients

- 4 cup of kale
- 4 tbsps. of olive oil
- 6 garlic cloves, finely chopped
- ½ tsp. of. salt

Method

- Preheat oven to 250F and line baking sheets with non-stick baking paper.
- Tear kale leaves into bite size pieces and transfer to a large bowl.
- Add the olive oil, garlic and salt and toss to combine.
- Lay the kale pieces in the baking sheets and bake for 15 minutes or until the edges are light brown.

Deviled eggs

Preparation time	5 minutes
Ready time	20 minutes
Serves	4
Serving quantity/unit	90 G / 3 ounces
Calories	160 Cal
Total Fat	15 g
Cholesterol	0 mg
Sodium	321 mg
Total Carbohydrates	8 g
Dietary fibers	1g
Sugars	0 g
Protein	3g
Vitamin C	1.36
Vitamin A	2.06
Iron	0.07
Calcium	0.1

Ingredients

- 4 large organic eggs, hard-boiled and peeled
- 1 tbsp. of mayonnaise
- 2 tbsp. of onion, finely chopped
- 1 garlic clove, finely chopped

- ¼ tsp. of salt
- ¼ tsp. of pepper
- ¼ tsp. of chili powder
- ½ tbsp. of parsley, finely chopped

Method

- Halve the eggs lengthwise, remove the yolk and transfer to a mixing bowl.
- Mash the yolk with a fork, add the mayonnaise, onion, garlic, parsley and seasonings and mash some more.
- Spoon egg yolk mixture into the halved egg whites and serve.

Raisin cookies

Preparation time	15 minutes
Ready time	25 minutes
Serves	5
Serving quantity/unit	40 G / 1 ounce
Calories	144 Cal
Total Fat	10 g
Cholesterol	0 mg
Sodium	22 mg
Total Carbohydrates	11 g
Dietary fibers	2 g
Sugars	8 g
Protein	5 g
Vitamin C	0
Vitamin A	0
Iron	0.04
Calcium	0.03

Ingredients

- 2/3 cup of almond flour
- 2 organic egg whites
- 1 tbsp. of coconut oil, melted
- 2 tbsp. of raw honey
- 2 tsp. of raisins

Method

- Preheat the oven to 350F.
- Line a baking sheet with non-stick baking paper.
- In a food processor combine the flour, egg whites, coconut oil and honey until smooth.
- Transfer to a mixing bowl and fold in the raisins.
- Scoop tablespoons of dough onto the prepared baking sheet and flatten each dough portion a little with your hands.
- Cook for 8-10 minutes or until golden.
- Remove from heat and let cool.

Grilled peaches with raw honey and lemon

Preparation time	5 minutes
Ready time	5 minutes
Serves	4
Serving quantity/unit	110 G / 4 ounces
Calories	73 Cal
Total Fat	0 g
Cholesterol	0 mg
Sodium	1 mg
Total Carbohydrates	19 g
Dietary fibers	2g
Sugars	17 g
Protein	1g
Vitamin C	0.14
Vitamin A	0.06
Iron	0.02
Calcium	0.01

Ingredients

- 4 peaches
- 2 tbsps. of raw honey
- 1 tbsp. of lemon juice
- 1 tsp. of cinnamon

Method

- Preheat an electric griller or a non-stick pan.
- Stir the honey, lemon juice and cinnamon in a small bowl until well blended. You can microwave this mixture for 15-20 seconds before serving.
- Halve and pit the peaches and grill covered with the cut side down for three or four minutes, or until tender.
- Serve two halves topped with the honey glaze and one tablespoon of cashews per person.

Baba Ganoush

Preparation time	15 minutes
Ready time	50 minutes
Serves	1
Serving quantity/unit	350 G / 12 ounces
Calories	133 Cal
Total Fat	5 g
Cholesterol	0 mg
Sodium	311 mg
Total Carbohydrates	22 g
Dietary fibers	11g
Sugars	9g
Protein	5g
Vitamin C	0.83
Vitamin A	0.72
Iron	0.09
Calcium	0.07

Ingredients

Baba Ganoush:

- 2 eggplants
- 4 garlic cloves, finely chopped
- 2 tbsp. of tahini
- 2 tbsp. of lemon juice
- ½ tsp. of salt
- ½ tsp. of pepper

Serve with:

- 1 carrot, cut into strips
- 1 red bell pepper, cut into strips
- 1 celery stalk, cut into strips

Method

Baba Ganoush:

- Preheat oven to 350F.
- Halve eggplants lengthwise and place them on a baking sheet with the cut side down. Poke the eggplants' peel with a fork in several places and roast for 30-35 minutes or until very tender. Let cool.
- Scoop out the eggplants meat from the peal. Transfer to a bowl and mash with a fork.
- Add the garlic, tahini, salt, pepper and lemon juice; mash some more.
- Serve the Baba Ganoush with the carrot, bell pepper and celery strips.

Apple and pear smoothie with collard greens

Preparation time	5 minutes
Ready time	5 minutes
Serves	4
Serving quantity/unit	200 G / 7 ounces
Calories	110 Cal
Total Fat	1g
Cholesterol	0 mg
Sodium	6 mg
Total Carbohydrates	28 g
Dietary fibers	6g
Sugars	18g
Protein	1g
Vitamin C	0.59
Vitamin A	0.16
Iron	0.02
Calcium	0.04

Ingredients

- 2 cup of apple
- 2 cup of pear
- ½ cup of banana
- 1 cup of strawberries
- 2 cup of collard greens
- 3 ice cubes

Method

- Combine all the ingredients in a food processor and pulse until smooth.

Roasted tomatoes

Preparation time	5 minutes
Ready time	60 minutes
Serves	4
Serving quantity/unit	130 G / 12 ounces
Calories	57 Cal
Total Fat	4 g
Cholesterol	0 mg
Sodium	297 mg
Total Carbohydrates	6 g
Dietary fibers	2g
Sugars	3 g
Protein	1g
Vitamin C	0.28
Vitamin A	0.21
Iron	0.03
Calcium	0.03

Ingredients

- 4 tomatoes, sliced
- 1 tbsp. of olive oil
- 3 garlic cloves, finely chopped
- ½ tsp. of salt
- ½ tbsp. of oregano

Method

- Preheat oven to 325F
- Combine all the ingredients in a large mixing bowl.
- Lay the tomatoes in an oven-safe dish and roast for 45-50 minutes.

Lunch

Sweet potato wedges with omelet muffin

Preparation time	20 minutes
Ready time	1h30m
Serves	4
Serving quantity/unit	335 G / 12 ounces
Calories	358 Cal
Total Fat	13 g
Cholesterol	206 mg
Sodium	605 mg
Total Carbohydrates	50 g
Dietary fibers	8g
Sugars	17 g
Protein	12g
Vitamin C	1.05
Vitamin A	8.91
Iron	0.16
Calcium	0.14

Ingredients

Omelet muffin:

- 5 organic eggs
- 3 tbsps. of grass-fed milk or almond milk
- ½ cup of red bell pepper, chopped
- ½ cup of zucchini, chopped
- 2 tbsps. of onion, finely chopped
- 2 tsps. of parsley, finely copped

- 1 tsp. of dill, finely chopped
- ½ tsp. of salt
- ½ tsp. of salt
- Sweet potato wedges:
- 8 sweet potatoes, cut into wedges
- ¼ tsp. of salt
- 2 tbsps. of olive oil

Method

Omelet muffin:

- Preheat the oven to 350F.
- Stir the eggs, milk, dill, parsley, salt and pepper in a large bowl until well blended.
- Prepare the filling combining the bell pepper, zucchini and onion in a bowl.
- Place a small amount of filling into the bottom of paper muffin liners, pour egg mixture into each cup of and bake for 20-25 minutes or until muffins are light golden brown.

Sweet potato wedges:

- Preheat oven to 250F and line baking sheets with non-stick baking paper.
- Place the potato wedges, olive oil, and salt in a large bowl and toss to combine.
- Lay the sweet potato pieces in the baking sheets and bake for 45 minutes or until a crispier texture is achieved.

Ham stuffed avocados

Preparation time	20 minutes
Ready time	30 minutes
Serves	4
Serving quantity/unit	260 G / 9 ounces
Calories	370 Cal
Total Fat	27 g
Cholesterol	120 mg
Sodium	1200 mg
Total Carbohydrates	19 g
Dietary fibers	9 g
Sugars	3 g
Protein	18 g
Vitamin C	0.42
Vitamin A	0.12
Iron	0.13
Calcium	0.06

Ingredients

- 2 avocados, halved and pitted
- 2 cup of organic ham, cubed
- 2 hard-boiled organic eggs
- 2 tomatoes, chopped
- 1 celery stalk, finely chopped
- 1 tbsp. of parsley, finely chopped
- ½ onion, finely chopped
- 3 tbsps. of lemon juice
- ½ tsp. of salt
- 3 garlic cloves, finely chopped
- ¼ cup of cashews

Method

- Scoop out the flesh from the peal of the avocados. Set aside the avocado's peel. Transfer the flesh to a bowl and mash with a fork.
- Add the remaining ingredients and stir to combine.
- Spoon the mixture into the avocado halves and serve.

Tuna patties

Preparation time	20 minutes
Ready time	55 minutes
Serves	4
Serving quantity/unit	260 G/ 9 ounces/ 3 patties
Calories	418 Cal
Total Fat	18 g
Cholesterol	77 mg
Sodium	397 mg
Total Carbohydrates	37 g
Dietary fibers	8g
Sugars	11 g
Protein	31 g
Vitamin C	0.56
Vitamin A	4.87
Iron	0.21
Calcium	0.16

Ingredients

- 2 ½ cups of sweet potato, cubed
- 2 cans of tuna in water
- 2 garlic cloves, finely chopped
- 1 onion, finely chopped
- 2 tbsps. of parsley, finely chopped
- 1 tbsp. of oregano
- ½ tsp. of salt
- ½ tsp. of black pepper
- 1 organic egg
- 1 cup of almond flour
- 2 tbsp. of lemon juice

Method

- Preheat oven to 350F.
- Drain the water from the tuna cans.
- Microwave sweet potatoes on High for 5 minutes or until just tender.
- Transfer to a mixing bowl and mash with a fork. Add the remaining ingredients, except for the flour, and stir to combine.

- Divide into 12 portions and shape each one into a patty with your hands.
- Coat the patties with the almond flour, remove the excess and lay them on baking sheets lines with non-stick baking paper.
- Cook for 10-15 minutes, flip and cook for further 10-15 minutes or until fully cooked.

Shrimp and pineapple salad

Preparation time	30 minutes
Ready time	40 minutes
Serves	1
Serving quantity/unit	343 G / 12 ounces
Calories	422 Cal
Total Fat	31 g
Cholesterol	124 mg
Sodium	470 mg
Total Carbohydrates	23 g
Dietary fibers	6 g
Sugars	14 g
Protein	19 g
Vitamin C	1.29
Vitamin A	0.83
Iron	0.25
Calcium	0.16

Ingredients

- 9 ounces of wild shrimp, peeled
- 8 cups of arugula
- 4 cups of Romaine Lettuce, shredded
- 4 cups of spinach
- ½ cup of basil, chopped
- 1 cup of pecan nuts
- 3 cups of pineapple, chopped
- 2+1 tbsps. of sunflower oil
- 3 tbsps. of lemon juice
- ½ tsp. of salt
- ½ tsp. of black pepper

Method

- Heat a non-stick pan and grill the shrimp with a little salt until it's fully cooked.
- Stir oil, lemon juice, pepper and salt in a small bowl until well blended.
- Place the greens in a large bowl, add the nuts, pineapple and shrimp. Toss to combine.
- Add the lemon dressing just before serving.

Turkey wrap

Preparation time	25 minutes
Ready time	40 minutes
Serves	4
Serving quantity/unit	380 G / 13 ounces /2 wraps
Calories	331 Cal
Total Fat	14 g
Cholesterol	42 mg
Sodium	1364 mg
Total Carbohydrates	36 g
Dietary fibers	7g
Sugars	20 g
Protein	19 g
Vitamin C	0.37
Vitamin A	2.03
Iron	0.18
Calcium	0.1

Ingredients

- 12 ounces of grass-fed turkey breast
- 8 large romaine lettuce leaves
- 6 tbsps. of raisins
- 2 cups of cucumber, cubed
- 2 cups of tomato, chopped
- 2 cups of carrot, grated
- 1 onion, finely chopped
- ½ cup of olives, sliced
- 6 tbsps. of mayonnaise
- 4 tbsps. of flax seed
- ¼ tsp. of salt
- ½ tsp. of pepper

- 1 tsp. of rosemary

Method

- Season the turkey with salt and rosemary and grill it in a non-stick skillet.
- Remove from heat, let cool and cut them into small pieces
- Spread the insides of the lettuce leaves evenly with the mayonnaise.
- Distribute the tomato, carrot, cucumber, onion, olives and flax seeds evenly among the prepared leaves.
- Top with the turkey and sprinkle with pepper.
- Wrap the lettuce and serve.

Crustless ham, asparagus and sun-dried tomato quiche

Preparation time	20 minutes
Ready time	1h10m
Serves	4
Serving quantity/unit	290G / 10 ounces / 2 slices
Calories	276 Cal
Total Fat	17 g
Cholesterol	274 mg
Sodium	1004 mg
Total Carbohydrates	14 g
Dietary fibers	3 g
Sugars	6 g
Protein	19 g
Vitamin C	0.79
Vitamin A	0.31
Iron	0.13
Calcium	0.08

Ingredients

- 1 ½ cups of organic ham
- 1 ½ cups of broccoli, chopped
- ¼ cup of sun dried tomatoes, finely chopped
- 3 tbsps. of onion, finely chopped
- 1 tbsp. of olive oil
- 6 organic eggs, beaten
- 1 ¾ cups of almond milk

- ¼ tsp. of salt
- 1 tsp. of oregano
- 1 tsp. of rosemary, finely chopped
- ½ tsp. of pepper

Method

- Preheat oven to 350F.
- Heat the oil in a non-stick skillet, add the onion and cook until translucent.
- Season with salt and pepper; add the broccoli and cook for 10 minutes. Add one or two tablespoons of water if necessary.
- Add the ham and cook for further 5 minutes. Remove from heat and combine with the tomato.
- Combine the eggs and milk in a mixing bowl.
- Line an oven-safe dish with non-stick baking paper, distribute the ham mixture evenly in the bottom of the dish and sprinkle with the herbs.
- Pour egg mixture into the oven-safe dish.
- Bake in for 30-35 minutes or until light golden brown.

Cucumber and salmon rolls

Preparation time	5 minutes
Ready time	5 minutes
Serves	4
Serving quantity/unit	335 G / 10 ounces
Calories	253 Cal
Total Fat	15 g
Cholesterol	45 mg
Sodium	675 mg
Total Carbohydrates	15 g
Dietary fibers	2 g
Sugars	6 g
Protein	16 g
Vitamin C	0.16
Vitamin A	0.53
Iron	0.07
Calcium	0.06

Ingredients

- 3 cucumbers
- 9 ounces of wild salmon
- 2 tbsps. of capers
- ¼ cup of olives, sliced
- 5 tbsps. of mayonnaise
- ½ cup of grated carrot
- ½ tsp. of salt

Method

- Combine the capers, olives, mayonnaise, carrot and salt in a mixing bowl.
- Thinly slice the cucumbers lengthwise with a vegetable peeler or mandolin.
- Spread a small amount of the mayonnaise dressing on one side of each cucumber slice and arrange the salmon on top of it.
- Roll up the cucumber slices and serve.

Dinner

Sweet and sour chicken and vegetables stir fry

Preparation time	15 minutes
Ready time	45 minutes
Serves	4
Serving quantity/unit	420 G / 15 ounces
Calories	428 Cal
Total Fat	13 g
Cholesterol	96 mg
Sodium	427 mg
Total Carbohydrates	45 g
Dietary fibers	5 g
Sugars	34 g
Protein	38 g
Vitamin C	2.15
Vitamin A	1.67
Iron	0.14
Calcium	0.09

Ingredients

- 1 pound of grass-fed chicken breast, cubed
- 1 onion, chopped
- 3 garlic cloves, chopped
- 1 ½ cups of carrot, sliced
- ¾ cup of green bell pepper, chopped
- ¾ cup of red bell pepper, chopped
- 1 ½ cups of cabbage, chopped

- 1 ½ cups of broccoli, chopped
- 2 cups of pineapple, chopped
- ½ cup of 100% pure, unsweetened, pineapple juice
- 2 tbsps. of olive oil
- 4 tbsps. of raw honey
- ½ tsp. of salt
- ½ tsp. of pepper
- ½ tsp. of chili powder

Method

- Combine the honey and pineapple juice in a mixing bowl; set aside.
- Heat the olive oil in a large non-stick pan. Add the onions and garlic and cook until it's translucent.
- Add the meat and cook for 7-10 minutes stirring occasionally.
- Add the carrots, bell peppers, cabbage and broccoli, season with salt and cook for 5-7 minutes.
- Add the pineapple, pepper and chili powder; cook for further 8 minutes.
- Set the heat to low, add the honey and pineapple juice mixture, stir and let simmer for 5 minutes.

Salmon with sun-dried tomato and lemon and kale chips

Preparation time	15 minutes
Ready time	1 hour
Serves	4
Serving quantity/unit	300 G / 11 ounces
Calories	524 Cal
Total Fat	39 g
Cholesterol	71 mg
Sodium	780 mg
Total Carbohydrates	19 g
Dietary fibers	4g
Sugars	2 g
Protein	31g
Vitamin C	2.89
Vitamin A	4.15
Iron	0.19
Calcium	0.22

Ingredients

Salmon:

- 1 pound of wild salmon fillets
- ½ tsp. of salt
- ¼ cup of sun dried tomato
- 3 tbsps. of olive oil
- 2 tbsps. of pecans
- 2 tbsps. of garlic
- ½ tbsp. of fresh oregano
- ½ tbsp. of fresh basil
- 3 tbsps. of lemon juice
- Kale chips:
- 8 cups of Kale
- 3 tbsps. of olive oil
- ½ tsp. of salt
- ½ tsp. of pepper

Method

Salmon:

- Cut 4 pieces of aluminum foil big enough to wrap the salmon covering it completely.
- Place each salmon fillet on top of an aluminum sheet.
- Combine the remaining ingredients for the salmon in a food processor and pulse until smooth. Distribute the mixture evenly on top of each fillet.
- Wrap up the aluminum sheets and place the wraps on a baking sheet.
- Bake for 25 minutes. Remove from the oven and carefully check is the salmon is fully cooked. If necessary, cook for further 10-15 minutes.

Kale chips:

- Preheat oven to 250F and line baking sheets with non-stick baking paper.
- Tear kale leaves into bite size pieces and transfer to a large bowl.
- Add the olive oil, salt and pepper and toss to combine.
- Lay the kale pieces in the baking sheets and bake for 15 minutes or until the edges are light brown.

Roasted chicken with parsnip puree

Preparation time	25 minutes
Ready time	3h30 minutes
Serves	4
Serving quantity/unit	410 G / 14 ounces
Calories	576 Cal
Total Fat	33 g
Cholesterol	96 mg
Sodium	1478 mg
Total Carbohydrates	50 g
Dietary fibers	8 g
Sugars	27 g
Protein	22 g
Vitamin C	0.83
Vitamin A	0.09
Iron	0.13
Calcium	0.08

Ingredients

Roasted chicken:

- 1 pound of chicken thighs
- ¼ cup of olive oil
- 4 tbsps. of parsley
- 1 tsp. of salt
- 1 tsp. of red pepper
- ¼ cup of raw honey
- ¼ cup of lemon juice
- ¼ cup of classic Dijon mustard (unsweetened)
- 1 small lemon sliced
- 3 garlic cloves, thinly sliced
- 3 onions, sliced

Parsnip puree:

- 1 pound of parsnips
- 2 garlic cloves
- 1 tbsp. of olive oil
- 2 tbsps. of almond milk
- ½ tsp. of salt

Method

Roasted chicken:

- Place the meat in a large bowl and set aside.
- In a small bowl, combine mustard, lemon juice, raw honey, parsley and garlic. Pour over the meat and marinate for at least 3 hours in the refrigerator.
- Preheat oven to 375F.
- Brush an oven-safe dish with half a tablespoon of olive oil and arrange the onion evenly on the bottom of the dish.
- Insert lemon slices between the skin and flesh of the chicken.
- Spread the remaining olive oil around the meat.
- Transfer the meat and juices to the prepared oven-safe dish, and sprinkle with salt.
- Cover with aluminum foil and roast for 25-30 minutes.
- Remove the foil. Lower the heat to 275F and cook for 20-25 minutes, or until meat is fully cooked, basting occasionally with the juices.

Parsnip puree:

- Wash, peel and slice the parsnips.
- Transfer to a pot, cover with water, and season with salt.
- Bring water to a boil and cook for 15-20 minutes, or until tender.
- Let cool, transfer parsnips to a food processor and reserve some of the cooking liquid.
- Add the olive oil, garlic and milk to the food processor and pulse until very smooth. Add a couple tablespoons of the cooking liquid to adjust the consistency if necessary.

Sweet potato and broccoli frittata

Preparation time	15 minutes
Ready time	40 minutes
Serves	4
Serving quantity/unit	380 G / 13 ounces
Calories	353 Cal
Total Fat	15 g
Cholesterol	205 mg
Sodium	573 mg
Total Carbohydrates	42 g
Dietary fibers	8 g
Sugars	5 g
Protein	15g
Vitamin C	1.3
Vitamin A	0.35
Iron	0.18
Calcium	0.11

Ingredients

- 5 organic eggs, beaten
- 3 organic egg whites
- 3 cups of sweet potatoes, cubed
- 1 tbsp. of olive oil
- 4 tbsps. of almond flour
- 1 onion, diced
- ¼ tsp. of salt
- ¼ tsp. of pepper
- ¾ cup of water
- 1 ½ cups of broccoli, chopped
- ¾ cup of red bell peppers, chopped
- ½ cup of sliced black olives, sliced
- ¼ cup of fresh parsley, finely chopped
- ½ cup of almond milk
- ½ tsp. of paprika
- ¼ tsp. of ground coriander
- ¼ tsp. of sea salt
- ¼ tsp. of black pepper

- ¼ tsp. of chili powder

Method

- Combine the eggs, whites and milk in a large mixing bowl and season with the paprika, coriander, black pepper and chili powder. Set aside.
- Heat the oil in a large skillet, add the onion and cook until translucent.
- Add the sweet potato, broccoli, bell peppers and a ¼ cup of water. Season with salt and cook for 15-20 minutes, or until tender, stirring occasionally. If necessary, add a little more water, but no more than a couple tablespoons at a time.
- Add the olives and distribute mixture evenly in the skillet.
- Pour the egg mixture over.
- Cook for 4 minutes or until eggs set, turn and cook the other side.

Chicken breast with honey and balsamic vinegar dressing and sautéed asparagus

Preparation time	20 minutes
Ready time	4 hours
Serves	4
Serving quantity/unit	270 G / 17 ounces
Calories	328 Cal
Total Fat	17 g
Cholesterol	73 mg
Sodium	644 mg
Total Carbohydrates	19 g
Dietary fibers	3 g
Sugars	15 g
Protein	27 g
Vitamin C	0.15
Vitamin A	0.18
Iron	0.18
Calcium	0.04

Ingredients

Chicken breast:

- 1 pound of grass-fed chicken breasts
- ½ tsp. of salt
- 1 tbsp. of Bay Leaf, crumbled
- 1 garlic clove, chopped
- 2 tbsps. of olive oil
- 3 tbsps. of balsamic vinegar
- 3 tbsps. of raw honey

Asparagus:

- 1 pound of asparagus
- 2 tbsps. of olive oil
- 4 garlic cloves, finely chopped
- ½ tsp. of salt

Method

Chicken breast:

- In a large bowl, combine the oil, balsamic vinegar, raw honey, garlic, and bay, and whisk.
- Add the chicken and marinate for 3 hours in the refrigerator
- Preheat oven to 350F.
- Transfer the chicken and juices to an oven-safe dish and sprinkle with salt.
- Cook the meat in the oven for 30-40 minutes, until fully cooked, basting occasionally with the juices.

Asparagus:

- Put enough water to cook the asparagus in a large pot, season with salt and bring it to a boil.
- Add the asparagus and cook for 2 or 3 minutes.
- Remove from heat and drain the water.
- Heat the oil in a large skillet, add the garlic and cook for half a minute.
- Add the asparagus and cook them for another 2 minutes.

Tuna stuffed eggplant

Preparation time	15 minutes
Ready time	1h10m
Serves	4
Serving quantity/unit	510 G / 18 ounces
Calories	362 Cal
Total Fat	14 g
Cholesterol	42 mg
Sodium	890 mg
Total Carbohydrates	36 g
Dietary fibers	15g
Sugars	13 g
Protein	29g
Vitamin C	0.38
Vitamin A	0.06
Iron	0.19
Calcium	0.18

Ingredients

- 2 large eggplants
- 2 cups of parsnips, cubed
- 1 onion, finely chopped
- 2 cans tuna in water
- ½ cup of organic tomato sauce
- ½ tbsp. of oregano
- ½ tsp. of white pepper
- 1 tbsp. of olive oil
- 3 garlic cloves, finely chopped
- ½ tsp. of salt
- 1/3 cup of almond flour
- ½ tbsp. of oregano
- ½ tbsp. of parsley
- ¼ tsp. of white pepper
- ½ tsp. of salt
- ¼ cup of parmesan cheese

Method

- Halve the eggplants lengthwise. Scoop out the flesh from the skin and reserve the skins.
- Cut the eggplants' flesh into small pieces, set aside.
- Drain the water from the tuna cans.
- Preheat the oven to 375F.
- Heat the oil in a skillet, add the onion and garlic and cook until the onion is translucent.
- Add the parsnips, eggplant meat and season with salt, oregano and pepper. Cook for 3 to 4 minutes.
- Add the tuna, stir and cook for another 2 minutes.
- Pour in the tomato sauce and let it simmer for 10-15 minutes, until the filling volume is reduced and it acquires a thicker consistency. Remove from heat.
- In a small bowl, stir the flour, parmesan cheese, oregano, parsley and salt to combine.
- Place the eggplants halves in a baking sheet and scoop in the tuna mixture, distributing it evenly.
- Spread the almond flour mixture evenly on top and bake for 20-25 minutes or until light golden.

Baked trout with sautéed vegetables

Preparation time	20 minutes
Ready time	1h25m
Serves	4
Serving quantity/unit	530 G / 19 ounces
Calories	456 Cal
Total Fat	26 g
Cholesterol	0 mg
Sodium	710 mg
Total Carbohydrates	27 g
Dietary fibers	9 g
Sugars	9 g
Protein	28g
Vitamin C	2.4
Vitamin A	3.49
Iron	0.11
Calcium	0.13

Ingredients

Trout:

- 1wild trout (around 1 pound)
- 1 large onion, sliced
- 1 green bell pepper, chopped
- 1 cup of peeled tomatoes, chopped
- ¼ cup of olive oil
- ¼ cup of white wine
- Juice of one lemon
- 4 tbsps. of parsley, chopped
- 3 garlic cloves, chopped
- ½ tsp. of black pepper
- ½ tsp. of salt

Vegetables:

- 3 cups of broccoli, chopped
- 3 cups of carrot, chopped
- 3 garlic cloves, finely chopped
- 2 tbsps. of olive oil
- ½ tsp. of salt

Method

Trout:

- Preheat oven to 375 degrees.
- Combine the olive oil, wine, lemon juice, parsley and black pepper in a mixing bowl.
- Brush the bottom of an oven-safe dish with a little of the olive oil mixture and arrange half of the onion on top.
- Carefully spread a couple tablespoons of the olive oil dressing all over the trout and place it on the prepared oven-safe dish.
- Sprinkle with salt.
- Pour the remaining olive oil over the fish and distribute the remaining onion evenly on top.
- Add the bell pepper and tomatoes.
- Cook in the oven for 30-45 minutes or until is fully cooked.

Vegetables:

- Heat the oil in a large skillet, add the garlic and cook for one minute.
- Add the vegetables, season and cook for further 15-20 minutes, or until the vegetables are tender. If necessary, add a couple tablespoons of water during the cooking process.

Desserts

Lemon custard

Preparation time	15 minutes
Ready time	55 minutes
Serves	4
Serving quantity/unit	101 G / 4 ounces
Calories	188 Cal
Total Fat	13 g
Cholesterol	180 mg
Sodium	109 mg
Total Carbohydrates	13 g
Dietary fibers	1g
Sugars	10 g
Protein	7g
Vitamin C	0.15
Vitamin A	0.08
Iron	0.06
Calcium	0.06

Ingredients

- ¼ cup of lemon juice
- 1 tbsp. of lemon rind
- 4 organic eggs, yolks and whites separated.
- 4 tbsps. of grass-fed milk or almond milk
- 2 tbsps. of raw honey
- 3 tbsps. of almond flour
- 2 tbsps. of clarified butter

- 1 tsp. of cinnamon

Method

- Preheat oven to 350F.
- Grease four ramekins.
- Beat the egg yolks and remaining ingredients, except the whites, with an electric mixer.
- Beat the egg whites until stiff and carefully fold them into the yolk mixture.
- Pour the batter into the prepared ramekins and place them on a baking pan. Fill ¼ of the baking pan with hot water.
- Bake for 30-40 minutes, or until its set in the middle.

Pineapple mouse

Preparation time	15 minutes
Ready time	12 hours
Serves	4
Serving quantity/unit	110 G / 4 ounces
Calories	130 Cal
Total Fat	4 g
Cholesterol	164 mg
Sodium	63 mg
Total Carbohydrates	16 g
Dietary fibers	1g
Sugars	14 g
Protein	8g
Vitamin C	0.34
Vitamin A	0.05
Iron	0.06
Calcium	0.03

Ingredients

- 1 cup of Pineapple
- ¼ cup of pineapple juice
- 1 packet of unflavored gelatin
- 2 tbsps. of raw honey
- 4 organic eggs, yolks and whites separated

Method

- Combine the yolks, pineapple, pineapple juice, gelatin and raw honey in a food processor and pulse until smooth. Transfer into a large bowl.
- Beat the egg whites until stiff and carefully fold them into the pineapple mixture.
- Cover and refrigerate overnight.

Banana and chocolate ice cream

Preparation time	5 minutes
Ready time	5 minutes
Serves	4
Serving quantity/unit	123 G / 4 ounces
Calories	225 Cal
Total Fat	15 g
Cholesterol	0 mg
Sodium	7 mg
Total Carbohydrates	30 g
Dietary fibers	8g
Sugars	16 g
Protein	4g
Vitamin C	0.14
Vitamin A	0.02
Iron	0.29
Calcium	0.03

Ingredients

- 3 frozen bananas
- 4 oz. of unsweetened dark chocolate

Method

- Place the chocolate in a food processor and pulse until finely chopped.
- Add the bananas and process until well blended.
- Serve immediately.

Mango and coconut pudding

Preparation time	5 minutes
Ready time	12 hours
Serves	4
Serving quantity/unit	105 G / 4 ounces
Calories	159 Cal
Total Fat	11 g
Cholesterol	1 mg
Sodium	26 mg
Total Carbohydrates	10 g
Dietary fibers	2g
Sugars	8 g
Protein	8g
Vitamin C	0.21
Vitamin A	0.07
Iron	0.05
Calcium	0.03

Ingredients

- 1 cup of mangos, peeled and pitted
- ¾ cup of coconut milk
- 28g/1 oz. of unflavored gelatin
- 3 tbsps. of grass-fed milk or almond milk

Method

- Place all the ingredients in a food processor and pulse until it is smooth.
- Transfer into a pudding dish and refrigerate overnight.

Melon and Basil Sorbet

Preparation time	5 minutes
Ready time	3-4 hours
Serves	4
Serving quantity/unit	281 G / 10 ounces
Calories	102 Cal
Total Fat	0 g
Cholesterol	0 mg
Sodium	34 mg
Total Carbohydrates	26 g
Dietary fibers	2g
Sugars	24 g
Protein	2g
Vitamin C	1.31
Vitamin A	1.33
Iron	0.03
Calcium	0.02

Ingredients

- 5 cups of melon
- 2 tbsps. of raw honey
- 1 cup of ice
- 1 tbsp. of basil
- ¼ cup of lemon juice

Method

- Combine all the ingredients in a food processor.
- Transfer to a metal container, cover and freeze for 3-4 hours or until it is slushy in the middle and hard on the edges.

Orange and chocolate cake

Preparation time	5 minutes
Ready time	5 minutes
Serves	10
Serving quantity/unit	80 G / 3 ounces
Calories	209 Cal
Total Fat	16 g
Cholesterol	65 mg
Sodium	174 mg
Total Carbohydrates	14 g
Dietary fibers	3 g
Sugars	9 g
Protein	7g
Vitamin C	0.05
Vitamin A	0.02
Iron	0.09
Calcium	0.05

Ingredients

- 1 ½ cups of almond meal flour
- 4 organic eggs, yolks and whites separated
- 2 organic egg whites
- 4 tbsps. of raw honey
- 8 tbsps. of raw cocoa
- 1 tbsp. of orange grind
- ¼ cup of orange juice
- ¼ cup of olive oil
- ½ cup of almond milk
- 1 tsp. of baking soda

Method

- Preheat the oven to 350°F.
- Combine the yolks, three tablespoons of oil and raw honey in a large bowl and add the milk.
- Mix flour with cocoa, baking soda, orange grind and cinnamon and add to the egg mixture.
- Beat the egg whites until stiff and carefully fold them in the cake batter.
- Grease a cake pan with the remaining oil and line it with non-stick baking paper.

- Pour in the batter and bake for 45 minutes or until a toothpick comes out clean.
- Set aside to cool but turn into a serving plate while still warm.
- Prick the top of the cake gently with a fork and spoon over the orange juice.

Paleo apple brownie

Preparation time	20 minutes
Ready time	1 hour
Serves	10
Serving quantity/unit	93 G / 4 ounces
Calories	166 Cal
Total Fat	12 g
Cholesterol	33 mg
Sodium	140 mg
Total Carbohydrates	16 g
Dietary fibers	2 g
Sugars	13 g
Protein	2g
Vitamin C	0.04
Vitamin A	0.02
Iron	0.03
Calcium	0.02

Ingredients

- 1 /3 cup of olive oil
- 2 organic eggs, yolks and whites separated
- ¼ cup of raw honey
- 3 apples, cut into small pieces
- 1/3 cup of pecan nuts, coarsely chopped
- 1 tsp. of cinnamon
- 1 cup of almond flour
- 1 tsp. of baking soda

Method

- Preheat the oven to 350°F.
- Combine the yolks, 4 tablespoons of oil and raw honey in a large bowl.
- Mix flour with the baking soda, and cinnamon and add to the egg mixture.
- Combine with the apples and nuts.
- Beat the egg whites until stiff and carefully fold them into the brownie batter.
- Grease a baking dish with the remaining oil and line it with non-stick baking paper.
- Pour in the batter and bake for 35 minutes or until a toothpick comes out clean.

Exclusive Bonus Download: Sprints And Marathons

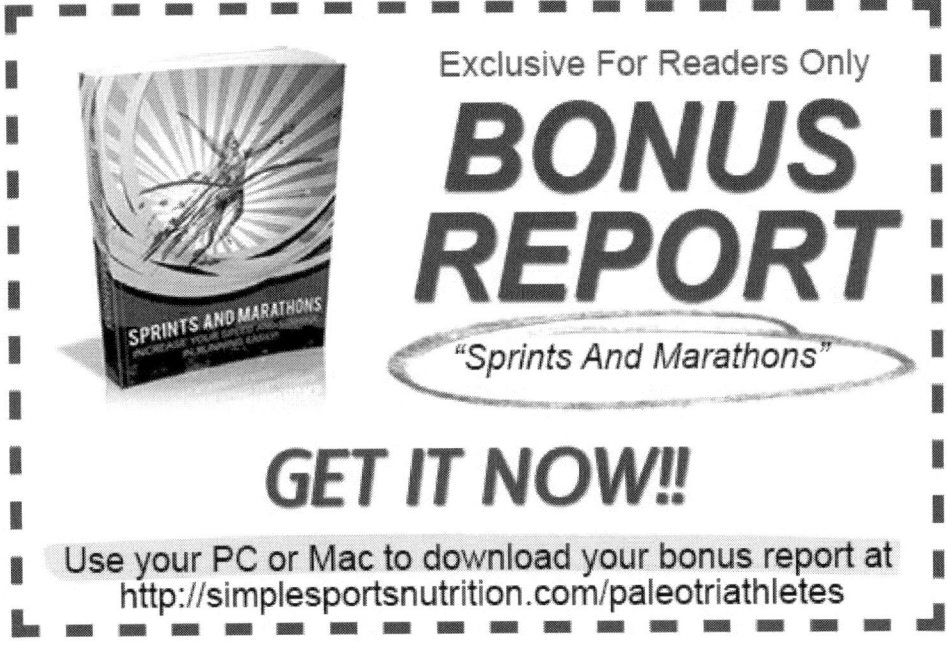

Download your bonus, please visit the download link above from your PC or MAC. To open PDF files, visit http://get.adobe.com/reader/ to download the reader if it's not already installed on your PC or Mac. To open ZIP files, you may need to download WinZip from http://www.winzip.com. This download is for PC or Mac ONLY and might not be downloadable to kindle.

Sure-fire Ways To Master Your Running Efforts!

This Book Is One Of The Most Valuable Resources In The World When It Comes To Getting Serious Results In Your Life!

Running is the act by which animals, including human beings, move by the power of the feet. Speeds may vary and range from jogging to a sprint. A lot of individuals compete in track events that place participants in a contest to test speed in a sprint or endurance in a marathon. The running mechanics are the same, but additional factors are very different in a marathon versus a sprint.

Consider this...

Whether your goal is to determine a fresh personal record in your next 5k, win your age bracket at the following charity run or qualify for a state or national contest, you may learn to run faster.

Are you ready?

Introducing… Sprints And Marathons

This powerful tool will provide you with everything you need to know to be a success and achieve your goal.

Who Can Use This Book?

- Life Coaches
- Runners
- Personal Development Enthusiasts
- Self Improvement Bloggers
- Business owners
- Internet marketers
- Network marketers
- Web Publishers
- Writers and Content Creators
- And Many More!

Visit the URL above to download this guide and start achieving your weight loss and fitness goals NOW

One Last Thing...

Thank you so much for reading my book. I hope you really liked it. As you probably know, many people look at the reviews on Amazon before they decide to purchase a book. If you liked the book, could you please take a minute to leave a review with your feedback? 60 seconds is all I'm asking for, and it would mean the world to me.

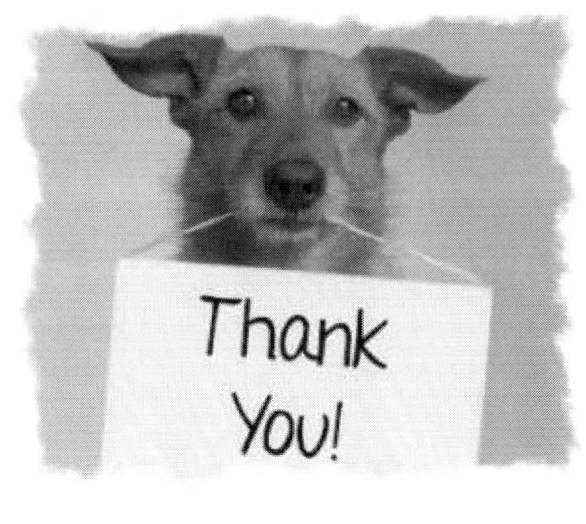

Books by Lars Andersen

The Smoothies for Runners Book

Juices for Runners

Smoothies for Cyclists

Juices for Cyclists

Paleo Diet for Cyclists

Smoothies for Triathletes

Juices for Triathletes

Paleo Diet for Triathletes

Smoothies for Strength

About the Author

Lars Andersen is a sports author, nutritional researcher and fitness enthusiast. In his spare time he participates in competitive running, swimming and cycling events and enjoys hiking with his two border collies.

Lars Andersen

Published by Nordic Standard Publishing

Atlanta, Georgia USA

NORDICSTANDARD
PUBLISHING

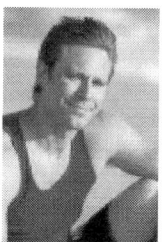

5794914R00042

Printed in Great Britain
by Amazon.co.uk, Ltd.,
Marston Gate.